Herbal Medicine:

30 Herbal Remedies to Heal Common Ailments

Table of content:

Introduction

You want to take control of your health.

The problem is there is too much information out there to sift through, and it's getting hard to tell the difference between fake remedies and proven ones. You looked up information online, in books, and have even asked owners and managers of health foods stores only to find you still have questions and wonder if the information is accurate. Wait no longer! I wrote this book with those concerns in mind. I have taken the time to sort through all the information and combed through studies to find the most relevant information on herbal medicine. I also walk you through what you need to make your own remedies and how long they keep before you have to make them again. I even include any possible side-effects and interactions with prescription drugs. What are you waiting for?

Chapter 1 - An Introduction

Herbalism has been around for millennia. It started in ancient China by trial and error. This meant they tried different plants to test their effects and rushed to find an antidote when they would accidentally ingest a poison. Though this doesn't seem like the smartest to document herbs and their uses, it eventually developed into what Asia knows as Traditional Chinese Medicine, which they practice to this day. India founded and still practices Ayurdeva, and Europe has an herbal pharmacology. In this day age, many mainstream physicians will work with people who have chosen to take herbal supplements.

The philosophy behind herbalism is approaching illness from a holistic method, meaning the whole body is looked at and not just the illness. By treating the body, mind, and spirit as well as the illness as one, the body will generally heal faster. This will also mean changes to lifestyle, diet, and how you mentally feel while you are ill. When symptoms are addressed by a holistic physician, they will be treated in the opposite order in which they manifested. Holistic medicine is about finding the root cause of the illness, not just treating symptoms.

This is a concern for many who delve into taking herbal supplements or taking herbal remedies for the first time. There are a few things to keep in mind.

Your body knows what you need. Learn to listen to it.

Your body know what's best for you. If you are taking an herbal supplement at start having reactions like headaches, indigestion, or other things along those lines, this is your body's way of telling you it doesn't need it.

If you are allergic to one plant in the family, be careful with other in the same genus/species.

Ragweed and Chamomile are related. This means if you are allergic to the weed, you may have reactions to the herb. Spend time looking to the herb you are interested in taking to make sure you are not allergic to its relatives.

If you are taking prescriptions for a medical condition, avoid herbs that work against it or will boost its potency.

An example of this would be Gingko Biloba, which has been proven to help improve memory. It is also a blood thinner. It is not recommended for you to take this herb if you are on medication to either thin the blood or reduce plaque deposits in your blood vessels. This also goes for beta blocker prescriptions and any herbals that are recommended for migraines or anti-depressants.

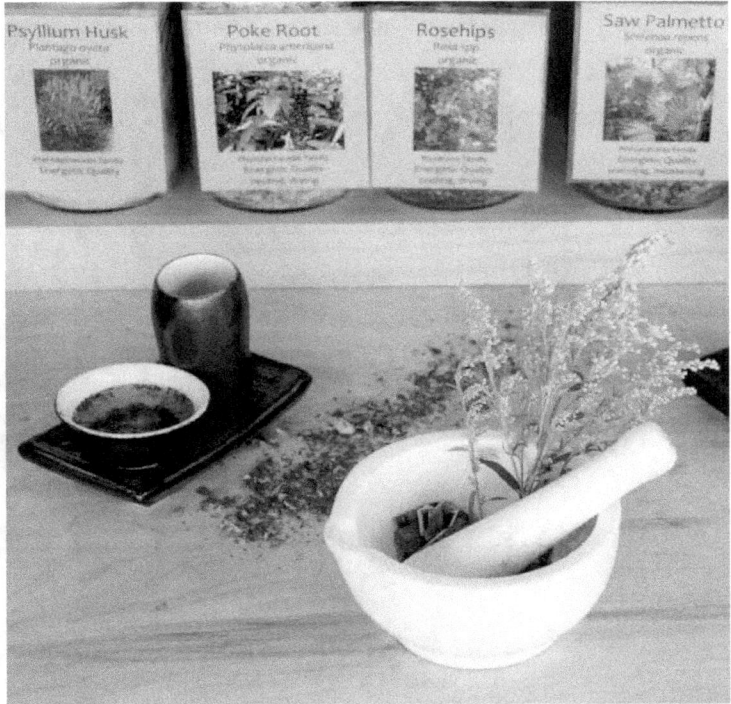

Before you start making your herbal remedies, you need to know all the different ways to make them. Here is a list which includes the shelf life of each.

● **Bolus**

This is a suppository and you can put it either in your rectum or your vagina, if you are female. These are generally made to directly apply the medicine to the affected area. This need to be used immediately.

How to make one:

In a double boiler add a tablespoon of coco butter and melt it. Add powdered herbs to the coco butter. Use aluminum to shape it into a bullet. Place it in the freezer to set. Insert the bolus and leave overnight.

• Capsules

This is the most common way for people to take remedies and supplements. These can keep their potency for up to two years.

To make them:

Mix the powdered herbs you wish to put in the capsules in a mixing bowl. Use a capsule making tool you can find online. Store them in a bottle with a tight lid in cool, dry place.

• Compress

This employs heat to help speed the healing properties of the ready to the injured area. They need to be used immediately.

How to make/use a compress:

Place 1/2 cup of herbs in a pot and three cups of water. Bring the water to a boil and simmer for an hour. Pour into a bowl and while still hot enough to place on the injured area, moisten a clean cloth and place on the injured area. As the compress cools change it out.

- **Decoction**

This is a type of tea which uses the roots, bark, and stems of the herb. For immediate use.

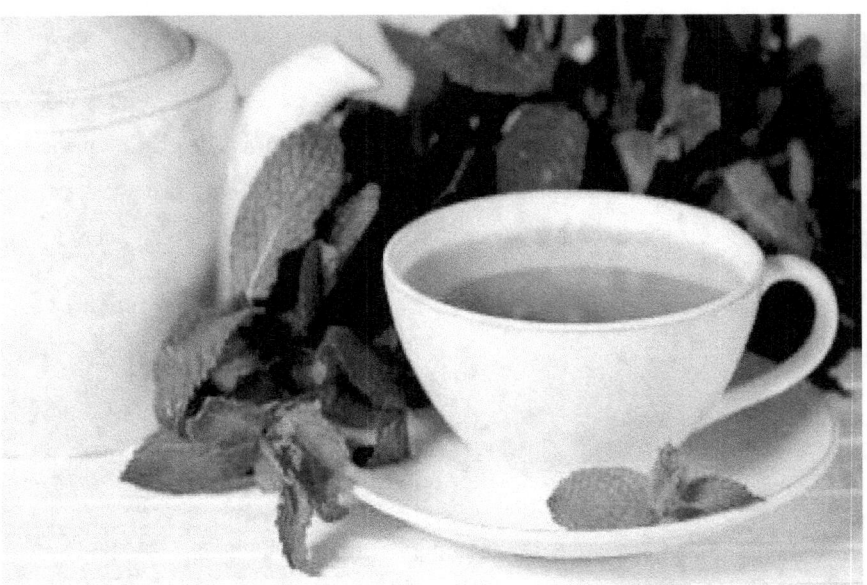

How to make one:

Therapeutic dose:

Use 1 tablespoon per each 6 ounce cup of water.

Maintenance dose:

Use 1 teaspoon per each 6 ounce cup of water.

Add the herbs to boiling water and boil for twenty minutes. Strain the plant matter out and add honey and lemon as needed.

• Extracts

This is a more potent preparation as far as this list is concerned. These are made by adding your herbs of choice to a solvent, letting the solvent leech the medicinal properties of herb out of the plant(s). You can either rub the extract on your skin or add up to 15 drops in a drink of your choice. Extracts last up to a year before losing potency.

How to make one:

You can use either four ounces of dried herbs or eight ounces of fresh, bruised (or mashed) herbs into a jar with a tight lid. Add to them one pint of either vinegar, alcohol, or rubbing alcohol. Shake the bottle twice a day for four days if the herbs you use are powdered or dry, and shake twice for fifteen days if you are using cut or whole fresh herbs.

• Hydrotherapy

This is an bath to which and strong herbal tea is added. This is commonly used for circulatory problems, skin problems, and to help detox.

How to make an herbal bath:

In a large stock pot, add one ounce of herbs. Fill the pot half-way. Bring the water to a boil and then simmer for twenty minutes. Strain out the herbs and add the tea to running water as you fill your bath.

• Infusion

This is a type of tea which uses the flowers and leaves of the herb.

To make an infusion:

Follow the directions for a decoction, but only boil for ten minutes.

• Oils

Herbal oils can be used both medicinally and for culinary purposes to add flavor to food. In herbal medicine, they are used for massage purposes.

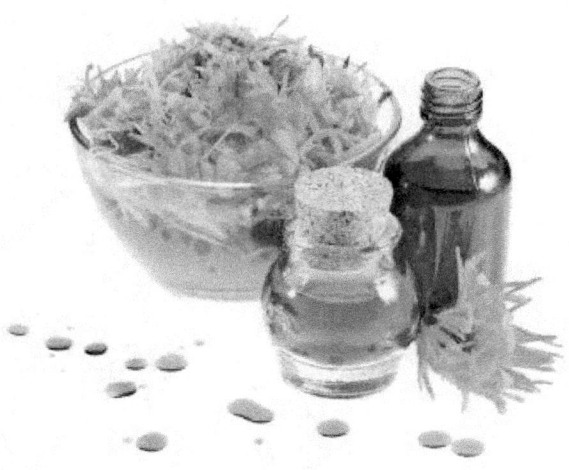

An herbal oil's shelf life is dependent on the oil you use to make it. Olive oil lasts the longest, but Sweet Almond is more commonly used and has a shelf life of six months to a year.

How to make an herbal oil:

Two ounces of an herb is added to one pint of oil. Sit the bottle, which should have a tight lid, in a warm place for four days. You can then strain the oil out for use. I quicker way of doing it is to use the same ratio and place the mixture into a crock pot on low overnight.

• Ointments

Ointments are thick and will stay on the skin for a longer period of time to help with minor injuries like bruises, bumps, sore muscles, and even rashes. They will keep for up to two years.

How to make an ointment:

You will need either Vaseline or non-petroleum jelly. Add two heaping tablespoons of the herbs to 1/2 a cup of the jelly. Heat on medium heat, stirring occasionally for twenty minutes. Strain the herbs out and place in a tightly lidded jar after it has cooled.

Poultices

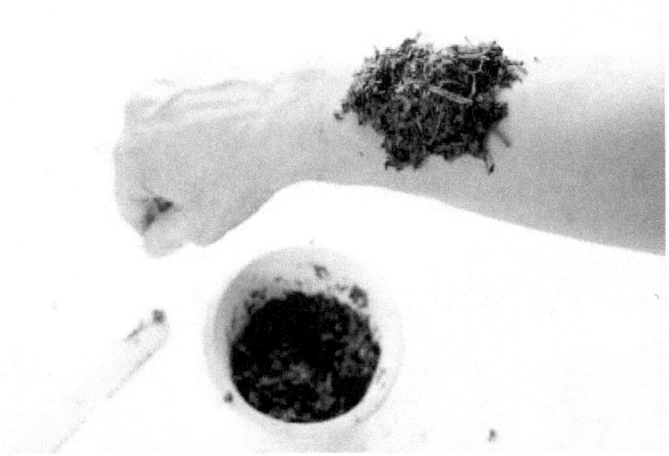

This is like a mask for your wound or injury. It is a thick mass of moistened herbs placed directly on the affected area. It is used in cases of bruising, insect bites, sprains and strains to keep the herbs in place for a long period of time. They can be applied either hot or cold but must be used as soon as they are made.

How to make a poultice:

Take an amount of herbs equal to the size of the area you wish to place the poultice. You can then mix in either hot water or herbal tea until it forms a thick paste. Powdered herbs are normally best for this. When it is still hot, but not hot enough to burn, place it on the affected area.

Powders

These are not commonly made it home due to a grinding process that can be tedious, but this is the preparation used in capsules, ointments at times, and also poultices.

Salves

These are like ointments because they are thick, but they are made completely different from their petroleum based counter part. Salves have a shelf life of about a year.

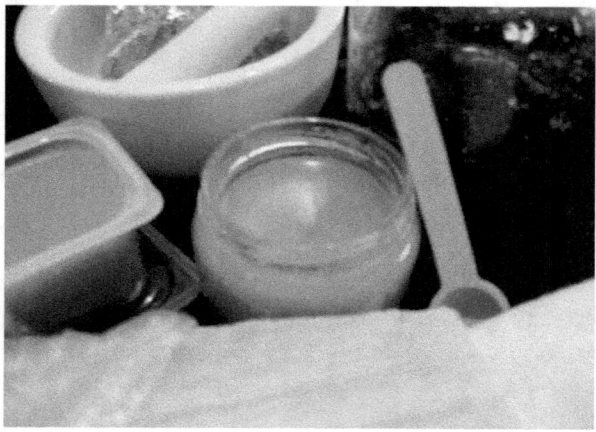

How to make salves:

You will need one cup of oil, 1/8 cup of beeswax beads and 1/4 cup of herbs. Make an herbal oil using the instructions for the crock pot. The next day, in a double boiler add the beeswax and melt. Stir in the oil without the herbs and place in a container with a tight lid. Apply to the affected area up to three times a day.

Syrups

These are good for stubborn colds, coughs, and even digestive problems. These keep for up to one week in the refrigerator.

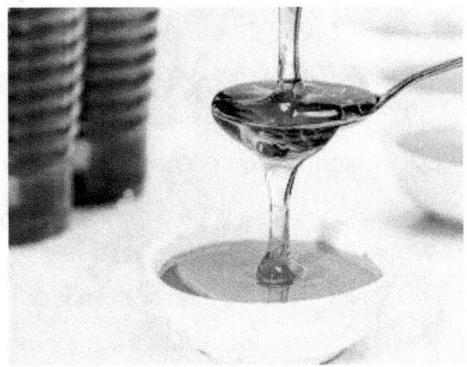

How to make a syrup:

Place 2 ounces of herbs in a stock pot and add one quart of water. Bring to a boil and let simmer until only a pint of water is left.

In a bottle or mixing container, place two ounces of either raw honey or vegetable glycerin. Strain out the herbs from the water and add the decoction to the honey or glycerin. Put a tight lid on it.

Tinctures

This are powerful concentrations of herbs made with alcohol in stead of water or vinegar. These are used in small doses and normally mixed in warm drinks for a more therapeutic kick. They can keep for up to two years.

How to make a tincture:

Add four ounces of herbals to a pint of either brandy or vodka. If you do not drink, you can add the herbs to boiled apple cider vinegar that has not been filtered. Allow the tincture to steep for up to four weeks, shaking every few days to mix the tincture well. You can strain out the herbs, but it is often not needed.

As you can see, there are a lot of ways to make and use herbs to treat injuries and illnesses. Which ones to make generally depend on the illness or injury and can be made using what you already have in your kitchen.

From a teacher to a mechanic, to do a job or hobby correctly, you need the proper tools. Making your own remedies is no different. Here is a list of what will be needed in order to make all the preparations above.

Glass or porcelain pots

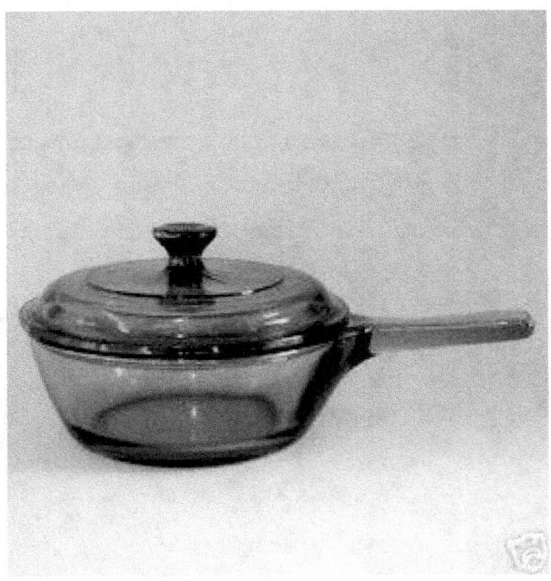

This may sound odd, but water and oil can leech the metal properties out of traditional pots and pans, often leading to a change in the way a preparation works. Glass and porcelain prevent the tainting of the mixtures.

Tea ball/reusable tea bags

These will often take a lot of the headache of straining herbs out for infusions, decoctions, syrups, and even herbal baths. You can find them online and even purchase one-use tea bags, both large and small, that you can use to keep your favorite blends. These can be sealed by using an iron or curling iron.

Double Boiler

You can also find these in glass. You can also rig your own by using a glass mixing bowl and placing it in a large pot that will hold it and add water to the pot. These are needed when you need to melt solid waxes and body butters without them touching the water.

Measuring spoons and cups

This are wonderful for measuring oils and herbs for smaller recipes.

Food Scale

Make sure this measures in ounces to make it easier for larger preparations like herbal baths, syrups and the like.

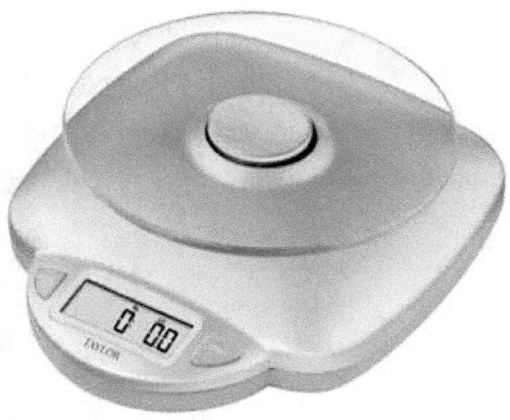

Strainers

Plastic strainers are good for this, but you have to make sure the plastic won't shrink when you pour hot liquids through them.

Glass bottles and jars

You can find these online for reasonable prices, and they can be a life-saver for storing your preparations from salves to syrups and tinctures.

Crock Pot

Just about everyone has one in their home for all-in-one meals, but they are great for steeping herbs in oils to make the herbal oil process a lot faster.

Mixing spoons

These can be bamboo or silicone, but they are needed for mixing preparations and helping to place ointments and salves into their containers.

Labels

This may seem like a weird thing to put on a list for herbal preparations, but you need to label your preparations and add the expiration dates so you don't use something that's out-of-date.

Recipe book/box

This is key to keeping track of all the preparations you make on a regular basis.

Now, let's get onto the body systems and remedies.

Chapter 2 - The Structural System

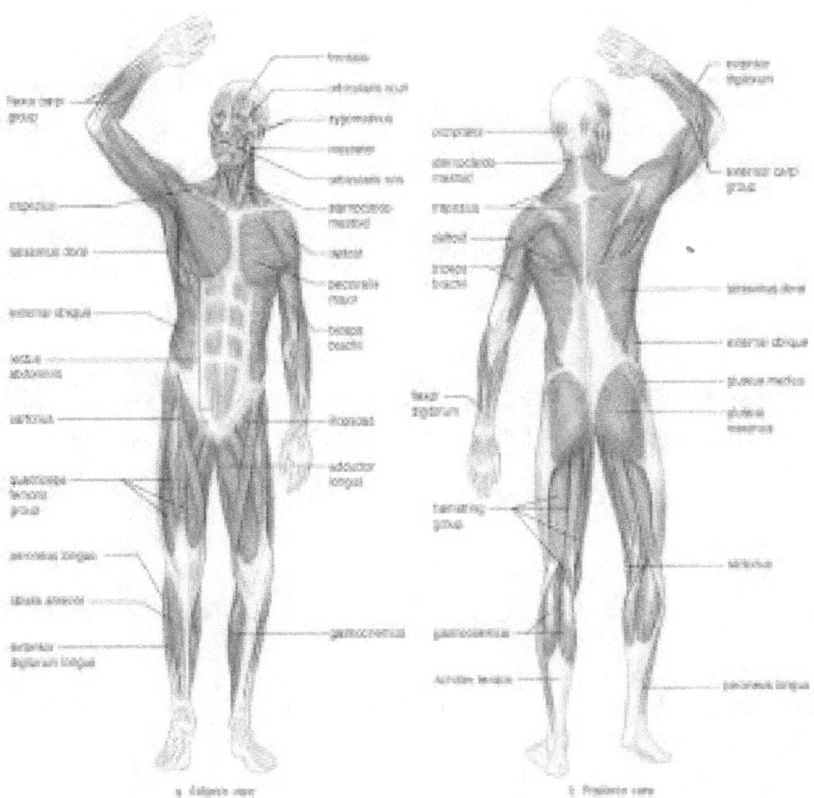

Your bones, joints, muscles, and skin all make up your structural system. Throughout our lives, depending on our activity level, we've all sprained an ankle, strained muscles, and even may have broken a bone. Most of us have had acne, but there are those of us who have had something we've tried to control but keep struggling with in terms of skin conditions.

Bruises

Everyday bumps and bruises can cause contusions, or bruises. There is a way to speed healing and get rid of the colorful reminder of having banged your body part.

Arthritis

This is a condition that attacks the joints and causes swelling, pain, and loss of movement/mobility. There are dietary restrictions to help prevent the swelling:

• Avoid the nightshade vegetables like tomatoes, potatoes, eggplant, and peppers.

• Keeping a diary of what you eat and how your arthritis reacts to what you eat can add to that list of foods to avoid.

Eczema and Psoriasis

These are skin conditions that are visible on the skin and can range from rashes that are cracked and bleeding to scale-like rashes that weep. Even though there are prescription medications that claim to bring these conditions under control, but they do it by suppressing the immune system, which can expose you to more serious diseases.

There are two ways to start being proactive when it comes to controlling these conditions:

• Get an allergy test. It have been proven, in some cases, these are allergic reactions to either environmental factors or food you eat.

• Manage your stress. This is easier said than done, but learning how to relieve and control stress will work wonders for controlling and, in some cases, relieve the condition altogether.

Bruise Salve

1 Cup of Sweet Almond oil (or Apricot Kernel oil if you're allergic to tree nuts)

1/8 Cup Beeswax

1 Tbsp *Arnica flowers*

(Really good for bruises)

1 Tbsp *Lavender Flowers*

(Good for Swelling)

(You can substitute Chamomile here)

1 Tbsp *Echinacea*

(Speeds healing)

Bruise poultice

2 Tbsp Arnica Flowers

Echinacea Tea

Joint Muscle Rub

6 Ounces of Sweet Almond Oil

2 Ounces of Olive Oil

2 Tbsp Juniper Berries

(Swelling and joint pain)

2 Tbsp Devil's Claw

(Joint pain and ligaments)

1 Tbsp Cinnamon

(Swelling and heating effect)

2 Tbsp Peppermint Leaves

(Cooling effect and anti-inflammatory)

Joint Herbal Bath

1/2 Ounce of Juniper Berries

1/2 Ounce of Lavender or Chamomile Flowers

Eczema Ointment

2 Tbsp Kelp

(Smooths the skin)

2 Tbsp Chamomile Flowers

(helps smooth skin)

2 Tbsp Echinacea

2 Tbsp Avocado Butter

(for extra moisture)

Psoriasis Rub

1/4 Cup Shea Butter

1/4 Cup Avocado Butter

(Both are excellent to toning and softening the skin and adding moisture)

2 Tbsp Lavender flowers

2 Tbsp Rose Petals

2 Tbsp Peppermint Leaves

1/4 ounce Aloe leaf

- Place the butters in a crock pot

- Add the herbs and steep overnight

- Strain out the herbs and place in a container with a tight lid.

- Let it cool before completely tightening the lid.

- Rub into the patches.

Chapter 3 - The Circulatory System

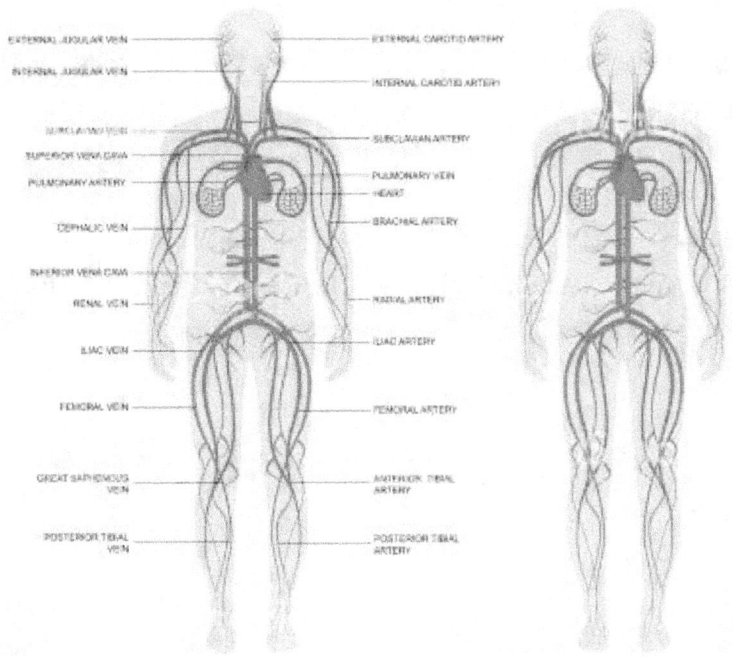

Your heart and blood vessels are the carriers of the oxygen that leaves you lungs. They also help you convey vitamins, minerals, and amino acids to your muscles. When your blood vessels start to clog, you can experience shortness of breath, low energy, and put your heart at risk because it's trying to work harder to get the blood to where it needs to go.

Heart disease and hypertension are two of the most prominent problems in our society. Taking care of your heart is very important for a healthy life.

Hypertension

Simply put this is very high blood pressure on a regular/daily basis. Left untreated, it can lead to heart attack and stroke.

As the skin condition above, relieving and learning how to manage stress can help lower blood pressure.

Changes in diet can do this as well. Even walking three times a week for at least twenty minutes can reduce your blood pressure. Here are a couple of recipes that can help without interacting with any medications you may be taking.

For a Weak Heart

Some people are born with congenital heart disease or a weak heart. This leads to them tiring easily and being short of breath.

Infusion for weak valves

1 tsp hawthorn berries crushed

(Highly recommended for a weak heart)

1 tsp night blooming cereus

(for valve malfunctions)

1 tsp catnip

(nervine)

Makes 1 therapeutic strength cup or 3 6-ounce regular strength cups.

Post-op Heart Attack Decoction

1 tsp hawthorn berries

1 tsp Dan Sheng Root

(Helps speed healing from heart operations)

1 tsp Lemon Zest (for flavor)

1 tsp Lavender flowers

(reduces swelling)

Hypertension

Just cooking with Basil and Cardamom can help to reduce your blood pressure. You can find these at any grocery store. Cooking with flaxseed is another way to help reduce your blood pressure.

Tea for Hypertension

Ginger tea is excellent for hypertension but if you can't handle the bite you can add Lavender and a little raw orange juice.

Blood Builders

These two recipes are to help strengthen blood vessels and for those who have low iron in their blood.

Iron Tea

1 tsp Red Raspberry leaves

1 tsp Red Clover flowers cut

1 tsp Butcher's Broom

Varicose Vein Bath

1/2 ounce Butcher's Broom

1/2 ounce Burdock Root

Chapter 4 - Digestive System

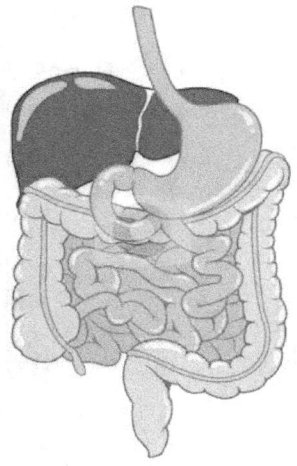

Upset stomachs, nausea, constipation, we've all experienced some sort of digestive issue. Stress, dietary choices, and even not getting enough fluids in your system on a daily basis can cause digestive issues. This does not discount actual intolerances, allergies, and diagnosed illnesses.

Heartburn

This is an over production of stomach acids to different degrees. Many antacids on the market can make this worse instead of better, leading to a complete dependence to the medication.

Here are some simple things you can do to help when it flares up:

• Parsley helps to curve heartburn. Chewing on a sprig will release the juice and stem the acid flow.

• Peppermint tea will help cool the burn.

Heartburn Tea

1 tsp Peppermint

(cools the core)

1 tsp Chamomile Flowers

1 tsp Lemon Balm leaves cut

(helps curve acid)

Drink cold

Marshmallow and Chamomile syrup

1 Ounce Marshmallow Root

(helps to absorb acids)

1 Ounce Chamomile Flowers

(calms the stomach)

2 Ounces Raw Honey

1 Tbsp every four to six hours.

Upset Stomach

This can be as small as an upset stomach to nausea and vomiting. Here are couple of things you can try:

- Chewing on a clove and swallowing the juice will alleviate nausea

- Putting a small amount of Allspice powder under your tongue will do the same.

Calming Tummy Tea

1 tsp Chamomile Flowers

1 tsp Peppermint leaves

1 tsp Fennel Seeds

(soothes the stomach)

Calming Tummy Syrup

1/2 ounce Peppermint Leaves

1/2 ounce Fennel Seeds

1/2 ounce Anise Seeds

1/2 ounce Lavender flowers

2 ounces raw honey

Chapter 5 - Nervous System

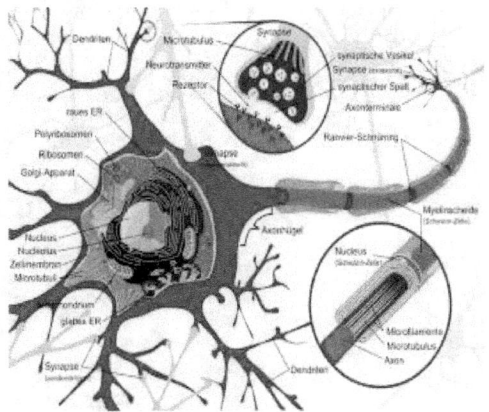

Made of our brain, eyes, spinal cord, and millions of synapses that fire off in order to deliver information to the brain the nervous system is truly a marvel, and many biologist have yet to unlock all its mysteries, but there are some ailments that are prevalent today which herbs to can help stem, if not help cure.

Alzheimer's Disease

Given a name in the late 80's this disease causes dementia in a patient, often reverting them back to child-like behavior and erasing memories of past experiences and even loved ones. There have been many reports of patients wandering off or family members getting in a car and driving only to not realize where they are.

Gingko Biloba has been tested, and in double blind studies has shown it can reverse early stages of Alzheimer's and lessen the severity of later stages.

Senility

This is quite different from dementia. Instead of wandering off or losing memories, it begins to present itself as being absent-minded and not able to recall things right away. This is simply due to the fact we need more B vitamins as we get older to help our brain function at the levels we are used to and for our nervous systems to function as they should.

Tea for concentration

1 tsp Peppermint leaves

1 tsp Gingko Bilboa

1 tsp Kelp (for B vitamins)

Extract for concentration

1 ounce Peppermint

1 ounce Kelp

1 ounce Gingko Biloba

1 ounce Gotu Kola

(Does the same thing as Gingko)

Anxiety can be debilitating. It can completely cripple someone leaving them unable to function. Here are couple of remedies that can help.

Nerve Tea

1 tsp Chamomile Flowers

1 tsp Catnip leaves

1 tsp Lavender Flowers

Herbal Bath

1/2 Ounce Lavender Flowers

1/2 Ounce Chamomile Flowers

Depression

Many people suffer from depression. It can take hours out of the day from your life by making you feel lethargic, and uninterested in everyday things. Just keep in mind, if you are bi-polar, you will have seek further advice from a licensed physician. The same goes for depression caused by chemical imbalances.

Saint John's Wort is the best herb to take for depression provided you are not already taking anti-depression medication.

There are headaches that can be a nuisance and there are migraines that can make chunks of your absolutely miserable with a spike is driven through your head. Thought they are still trying to figure out all the root causes of migraines there are few things you can do to help stave some of them off:

• Log smells, foods and other things that can trigger a migraine.

• High stress can also cause migraines.

You can help relieve stress by meditation, and listening to soothing music when you come home from a busy day.

Migraine Tea

1 tsp Feverfew

1 tsp Peppermint

Chapter 6 - The Glandular System

This is the system that can regulate everything from the metabolism to you hormones and everything in between. Even though the liver is generally considered part of the digestive system, I have put it here because of it's filtering abilities and how it aids the pancreas in regulating blood sugar levels.

Diabetes

This is a well-known disease which involves the pancreas. Insulin is created by the pancreas to regulate blood sugar, but when starts to malfunction, it can produce less and less, leading to higher levels of glucose in the blood. This can cause dizziness and fainting spells, mood swings, and in more severe cases diabetic comas.

Nopal can help regulate glucose levels, and Stevia, a natural sweetener that is 10x sweeter than sugar, can as well.

Blood Sugar Tea

1 tsp Juniper Berries

1 tsp Ginger

1 tsp Billberry

Blood sugar Capsules

Equal parts of the following herbs in powder form:

Juniper berries

Nopal

Billberry

Stevia

It is recommended that you constantly check your blood sugar level if you are already on medication for this to make sure you are not lowering your glucose levels to dangerous numbers.

Liver/ Gall Bladder

Your liver and gall bladder take the brunt of the abuse when it comes to filtering out any toxins in your system. From fats to alcohol and even artificial additives, these two glands work hard to make sure you will not get ill from toxicity, but when they are overworked, you can run into problems.

Detox Tea

1 tsp Milk thistle seeds

(excellent for detoxing the liver)

1 tsp Dandelion root

(good for liver and water retention)

Prostate

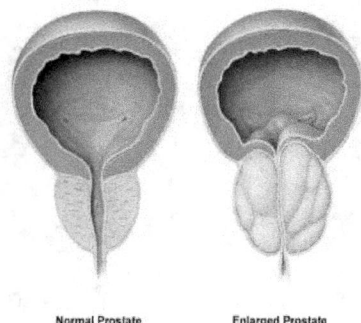

Normal Prostate   Enlarged Prostate

Prostate health is very important for men. Regular checks can lead to early detection for cancer and other prostate problems. There is also something you can take to maintain prostate health.

Saw Palmetto is the best supplement you take on a regular basis to maintain prostate health.

Menopause

The change of life can be hell on a woman. Here are a few suggestions you can try to make the transition to and the menopause itself easier.

Black Cohosh is the most popular, but it often does not work for all women.

Evening primrose can help with night sweats and hot flashes.

Wild Yam and Chaste Tree Berries are a wonderful combination for those that find the first two recommendations do work as well as they had hoped.

Chapter 7 - Keep Learning

There are a myriad more herbals out there than the ones I have mentioned in this book. Botanical.com is a great way to get started on your way to learning herbs. There are books which can continue your education as well. Today's Herbal, by Louise Tenney is a highly recommended start book for those wanting to learn more.

Experiment with different herbs and combinations to find what works best for you. You may even need to rotate supplements out from time to keep your body metabolizing different herbs and combinations. Your body can get used to them as time goes by.

Go onto online groups and forums to ask advice, learn about new herbs and expand your knowledge. You can even learn about essential oils and homeopathic remedies to compliment what you are already doing. You will be surprised what you can come up with when you have the right information and start mixing different herbs.

Conclusion

I hope this book answered questions that you had and didn't know you had. This book was meant to start you on your way to learning about a whole new field of natural health and taking control of your life, your body, and your health above all.

Please, be on the lookout for more books on natural health in this series, and as always, never stop asking questions.

www.ingramcontent.com/pod-product-compliance
Lightning Source LLC
Chambersburg PA
CBHW062026280526
45787CB00005B/2228